The 5-Second Cure

*Your Surprisingly Simple
Solution to Avoid Getting Sick
and Beat Disease Naturally*

By
K.D. Joseph

If you would like to contact the author with any questions please email:

kdjosephadvice@gmail.com

How to stop getting sick

THIS brief guide is going to show you a simple, uniquely effective way to avoid getting sick. It will help you substantially reduce the number of common colds and cases of the flu you get for the rest of your life.

In short, if you hate getting sick, you should read these suggestions.

The bonus of this guide, for the curious reader, is that it can also show you how to treat and cure more serious health problems in an easier way. The essence of this material contains deeper implications than just learning how to treat the common cold.

What I regard as the easiest, simplest and most effective way to become healthier has changed as the years have passed. The health advice I recommend to people has become less and less complicated – while, in my opinion, becoming more effective. This particular guide contains probably the easiest and most simple health tip I have ever encountered.

When it comes to personal health, many things we initially think are true turn out to be false, and ideas that might at first seem slightly absurd sometimes actually end up being the most effective long-term health solutions.

I was skeptical about the main ideas offered in this guide when I originally encountered them. They seemed too good to be true. But after doing some research, trying the ideas for myself, and then with clients, my thinking has completely changed in regards to their effectiveness.

The primary tip in here seems so easy that, like me, I doubt you'll believe it at first. It's a "secret" only because so few people actually believe that advice this simple could work as well as it does. Because it sounds so easy, some people will dismiss the advice before they even try it. I encourage you not to be one of those people.

What I'm about to share with you will make it so you hardly ever get sick. It will only take five seconds of your day, and is completely painless. Anybody can do it, and because of that, you should feel free to tell other people about it. It works well for anyone because it's essentially effortless.

So I really encourage you to use this easy health suggestion. You have nothing to lose, and a lot to gain.

The only other thing I should emphasize is that you should feel no pressure as you read this guide. Relax. Please don't try to be perfect in regards to your health. Just be you, which is perfect already, and you'll be more than fine.

You can't screw up this advice; I promise you. It's too easy to screw up. And it works. It really, really works. If you have questions or are confused, let me know. You can always email me at any time concerning the suggestions in this guide. I'm here to help if you want it.

Now onto the "secret" advice. To dramatically reduce common illnesses, you simply take high dosages of Vitamin D3 and Vitamin K2 daily.

And…that's it. When I said it was simple, I wasn't kidding.

This unexplored D3 and K2 vitamin combination can dramatically improve your health, and, at the very least, it will help you get sick far less often. It's so easy, safe, cheap and effective that it's a no-brainer. So try it.

I'll give you the specifics of approximately how much Vitamin D3 and Vitamin K2 you should be taking in a moment, but first I should tell you that, generally speaking, I'm not a vitamin person. I have never liked taking pills every day, let alone recommending them to others. Usually I think that kind of health advice is mildly absurd.

But, for whatever peculiar reason, the high dosage of Vitamin D3 and Vitamin K2 taken together works wonders. And ultimately I don't really care how something works, as long as it does work.

Vitamin D is a supplement you might already be familiar with. The "sunshine" vitamin makes sense on many levels. The most intuitive one is that the human species has thrived for tens of thousands of years by getting enough sun exposure. Humans do well physically by being exposed to the sun, it makes us feel good, and we get sick less often due to that exposure. That's why we're more likely to get sick in the winter instead of summer - we don't get enough sunlight.

Very few of us nowadays get enough sun exposure on our skin at any time of the year, especially with our over-zealous sunscreen usage. Therefore, it's worthwhile to supplement with Vitamin D3 tablets.

Vitamin D3 is generally regarded as a good vitamin to combat illness, particularly in the winter, although it's not explicitly promoted as such. Taking D3 alone – about 5,000 IU a day – helps combat the common cold and flu. 5,000 IU is a large, safe, appropriate amount for anybody over the age of ten to take daily.

D3 is cheap, and taking it has subtle financial advantages as well as health benefits. You end up not paying as much for cold and flu medicines. You won't miss as much work, and you no longer will have to worry about a bad cold ruining your ability to get things done. But obviously, these minor financial advantages aside, the real benefit of D3 is that you don't get sick and feel terrible as often.

Some of you might already be taking Vitamin D3 – but probably in a lower dosage than you optimally should be. 1,000 IU of D3 daily, for example, is better than nothing, but you'll see great improvements if you increase your regular dosage.

We should aim to usually be taking at least 5,000 IU of D3 daily. There's not a good reason to be taking less than that. Simply search online or go to a health food store to find many popular brands of 5,000 IU Vitamin D3 supplements.

Vitamin D3 does a lot more than just help promote a healthy immune and skeletal system. That's because D3 is not really a traditional vitamin, but a steroid hormone. This is good news, because D3 therefore helps your body effectively fight all types of diseases and ailments.

High dosages of D3 can dramatically help prevent, treat, and sometimes cure a wide array of serious health problems. These include psoriasis, obesity, diabetes, arthritis, multiple sclerosis, Alzheimer's, numerous types of cancers (including leukemia, breast cancer, colon cancer and lymphoma), autism and schizophrenia.

Do I have your attention yet? This is not a normal vitamin we're talking about.

You should be taking a *large* dosage of Vitamin D3 daily – at least 5,000 IU a day. Don't worry if you skip a day every now and then because it doesn't matter. Just get into the habit of taking it daily with a meal. Start taking advantage of Vitamin D now.

This guide, however, is not just about Vitamin D. It's about taking both Vitamin D3 and Vitamin K2 together on a regular basis.

I think there's a significant difference. Vitamin K2 is considered to be important in promoting bone density, coagulation and arterial health. These obviously sound like positive things. But what this really means, in relation to taking Vitamin K2 with Vitamin D3, is that the K2 will help the D3 assimilate into your body in the most effective way possible.

If you want your D3 supplementation to be as effective as possible, and avoid the common cold and flu, you should be taking K2 alongside your D3. It helps significantly, believe me.

Vitamin K2 comes in two supplemental forms, either MK-4 or MK-7. Both forms work well for the vast majority of people. Again, you can easily find and purchase these Vitamin K2 supplements online or at a health food store. I recommend taking a Vitamin K2 supplement once every day or two with a meal.

That's all there is to it, in a nutshell. We don't need to make it sound more complicated. Let's just keep it simple:

Take a large supplement of Vitamin D3 daily, at least 5,000 IU. Also take a Vitamin K2 supplement regularly so all the D3 is absorbed by your body in the best way possible. Take these supplements with a meal, not on an empty stomach. If you do this – and it only takes a few seconds a day – you will greatly reduce the number of colds and cases of the flu you get for the rest of your life.

It's also worth mentioning that if you feel a cold coming on, it is advantageous to take a very high dosage of D3 for a few days – like 20,000 IU to 50,000 IU daily – in order to counteract the illness. Be sure to take a few K2 tablets with all that D3. That will prevent many a cold from developing any further.

So, congratulations, you no longer have to be concerned about constantly getting sick. Pretty soon, many of you will forget that you even used to get sick with any type of regularity. I can tell you this is a huge relief. Congratulations on a job well done!

Now comes the "advanced" part involving the peculiar effectiveness of this Vitamin D3 and Vitamin K2 cocktail. If you were only interested in avoiding getting sick, feel free to stop reading. If you're curious in finding out a way to improve your health in a more substantial manner, I think you'll enjoy trying out what I'm about to describe in simple terms.

Using "advanced" Vitamin D3 and Vitamin K2 techniques

WHAT Vitamin K2 also enables us to do is to take much higher daily dosages of Vitamin D3 than we could safely take if we weren't supplementing with K2. Vitamin K2 allows Vitamin D3 to be absorbed properly in the body even at extremely high levels of supplemental intake. These huge amounts of D3 can enable substantial healing to occur, a level of heightened healing that otherwise might have been impossible if the D3 was taken without K2.

Without K2 you can take a significant daily dosage of D3 with zero long-term health concerns – say about 5,000 IU a day, to play it safe. But when you're daily supplementing with K2, you can substantially increase your D3 intake. Why would you want to do this?

If you have health issues you would like to try to improve or cure, taking a very large daily dosage of Vitamin D3 is probably the cheapest, easiest way to do it.

The best book on taking big dosages of D3 is Jeff Bowles' *"The Miraculous Results of Extremely High Doses of Vitamin D3."* It's a fascinating book, and it is how I first encountered the unusual concept of taking considerable amounts of Vitamin D.

The main point Bowles makes is that high dosages of Vitamin D3 have strangely effective curative powers. What does Bowles mean when he says high dosages? 20,000 IU to 100,000 IU of Vitamin D3 taken daily. That's a lot of D3! Bowles calls this "mega-dosing," and the idea would probably seem crazy – if it weren't so effective.

High dosages of D3 have shown to not only help, but actually cure and heal, many serious ailments. In the book Bowles shows that large dosages of D3 regularly cure seasonal depression, bone and joint pain, asthma, psoriasis, diabetes and heart disease. The real world case studies he provides are genuinely uplifting.

Also, interestingly, high dosages of D3 seem to be a great way to effortlessly lose weight. Many people seem to lose ten pounds or more over a relatively short period of time, just by taking a very high dosage of D3, and changing nothing else. Read that again. That's right, you can potentially lose a significant amount of weight just by taking a vitamin. It turns out that the "too good to be true" magic pill promise might be real – as long as the pill is Vitamin D3.

I think you should always be taking K2 with your D3, because it greatly helps D3 assimilate into your body. But if you want to try "mega-dosing," it's absolutely essential.

K2 is very important to take alongside large amounts of D3, because it solves any calcium/bone/arterial/heart issues you might potentially otherwise have by taking so much D3 alone. You can't overdose on Vitamin D3 if you take Vitamin K2 with it.

The general guidelines are to take approximately 100 mcg of MK-7, or 1,000 mcg of MK-4, for every 10,000 IU of D3 you ingest. You don't need to be exact by any means; the important thing is just for there to be sufficient levels of

K2 entering your body along with all that D3.

In other words, these are approximate daily intake guidelines to follow when you "mega-dose":

10,000 IU of D3 equals:
100 mcg of MK-7 or 1,000 mcg of MK-4

20,000 IU of D3 equals:
200 mcg of MK-7 or 2,000 mcg of MK-4

30,000 IU of D3 equals:
300 mcg of MK-7 or 3,000 mcg of MK-4

50,000 IU of D3 equals:
500 mcg of MK-7 or 5,000 mcg of MK-4

100,000 IU of D3 equals:
1,000mcg of MK-7 or 10,000 mcg of MK-4

Another thing worth mentioning is sleep. Getting ample sleep is essential if you're taking high dosages of Vitamin D3. We can all think of times when we were out in the sun all day. We often were exhausted by the early evening and needed a good night's sleep. Consider this while you are taking a very high dosage of Vitamin D3. Get plenty of sleep. Don't be afraid to sleep 10 to 12 hours a night if your body feels the need. This sleep will help you heal faster, and make you feel better.

I encourage you to read Bowles' book to get more insight into his recommendations and case histories involving Vitamin D. The information in it can legitimately help you improve your health – just by doing something that takes five seconds a day.

If you have questions regarding this material, or any general questions, feel free to email me at:

kdjosephadvice@gmail.com

Thanks for reading, and cheers to your health!

- K.D.

Breakfast is Bullsh*t

*How You Will Lose Weight and
Become Healthier by Skipping the
Most Important Meal of the Day*

Breakfast is the most overrated meal of the day.

In this short book you will see that if you want to be healthier, and lose unwanted weight, you should stop eating breakfast. There is simply no need to be eating in the morning, and your body will be grateful if you give up this unnecessary dietary habit.

If the idea of skipping breakfast for health reasons seems shocking to you, it won't be once you are finished reading this guide. The popular opinion of breakfast being the most important meal of the day is a myth. And if you skip breakfast for yourself over the next few weeks you will get to pleasantly experience this fact for yourself.

People get worried that they'll be detrimentally hungry if they start skipping breakfast, as if the lack of food in the morning will destroy their lives. After a few days of actually skipping breakfast, you'll realize how ridiculous a fear this is.

The truth is that in our modern culture, the vast majority of people overeat. Hunger is a mental thing, not a physical thing. Our human body is pretty incredible. Even as amazing as modern medicine is, our body is still usually its own best healer. But our body works best when we generally leave it alone and don't constantly overfeed it.

Hunger is mental in our culture.

It's worth remembering that. Be gentle and loving of your body, and try not to overeat. Then watch your health naturally improve without effort, simply by not interfering with your body's incredible, inherent healing powers. Assume health, and become healthy. If you follow these simple steps, and begin to feel yourself as already being healthy, then health will follow.

Not eating until you are truly hungry is a rather intuitive thing, when we're not unnecessarily neurotic about eating and food (all of us, unfortunately, can think of times when we have been neurotic about what we eat.) Skipping breakfast allows you the pleasure of not overeating, not overanalyzing what you eat, and a better enjoyment of whatever you do decide to eat.

Take advantage of this wonderfully simple eating model, there's little reason not to. The most important thing is not when you eat, but not overeating simply for the sake of it. Take breakfast, excess food consumption, and constantly worrying about your body out of the equation. You deserve better than that, and you'll be amazed how much better you feel when you begin doing it.

Start enjoying eating in a more meaningful way. If you can give this gift to yourself, your body will gratefully thank you, and you'll be rewarded with better health, naturally.